Wellness Wisdom for Women: Simple Self-care Strategies

By

Lilly Green

Dedication

This book is dedicated to all women seeking to nourish their minds, bodies, and spirits. May you find inspiration in these pages for a lifestyle of self-care and natural wellness that honors your beautiful, unique self.

Foreword

We all could use gentle reminders to slow down and care for ourselves. This book provides simple, practical guidance to help women thrive in body, mind, and spirit. Drawing on the author's journey to well-being, it empowers readers to craft a self-care routine with easy home remedies, stress relief practices, nutritious recipes, and more. A must-read for your healthiest, happiest self!

-Dr. Sheila Davis, Functional Medicine Practitioner

Copyright ©

Table of contents

About the author

Meet Lilly Green, Wellness Author, and

Advocate. Lilly Green also known as (Dr. Emily Turner) is an author, speaker, Herbs partitionist and natural wellness advocate who empowers women to care for their whole selves. After struggling with anxiety and exhaustion in her corporate career, Olivia made major lifestyle changes and found her true passion in promoting holistic well-being.

She left her stressful job and enrolled in massage therapy and aromatherapy programs. Olivia saw firsthand how small daily practices like meditation, preparing nutritious foods, and using natural remedies can transform wellness. She wanted to share these insights with others.

Lilly began teaching and leading wellness workshops for women in her community. She launched a successful blog featuring stress relief tips, healthy recipes, and DIY spa treatments. Her weekly wellness newsletter gained thousands of dedicated readers.

After requests for a comprehensive guide, Olivia wrote her first book "Natural Wellness Tips for Women" sharing her journey along with advice on managing stress, nourishing your body, natural beauty remedies, and more. She has since authored 3 more bestselling books on self-care, healthy cooking, and mindfulness.

When she isn't writing, Olivia enjoys hiking, cooking, reading, and spending time with her family and tending her garden. She continues   to teach workshops and speak at wellness conferences. Olivia's mission is to help busy women slow down, care for themselves, and cultivate inner calm.

I'm so glad you picked up this book! I wrote Natural Wellness Tips for Women to share the self-care practices that have transformed my life in hopes that they can help you thrive too. We all have so many responsibilities and pressures these days. It's easy to put ourselves last, depleting our health and happiness. My goal is to provide simple yet effective ways to nourish your body, mind, and spirit every day.

In this book, you'll learn techniques I've used myself to manage stress, make home-cooked meals, pamper yourself with natural beauty remedies, and support overall well-being. These small steps don't require drastic lifestyle overhauls - they can

become part of your daily self-care routine. When we care for ourselves, we become our best selves. I hope these natural wellness tips help you slow down, relax, and remember to make yourself a priority.
Now let's begin the journey!

Introduction

Welcome, dear reader, to a transformative journey of self-care and natural wellness. In our busy modern lives filled with never-ending responsibilities and pressures, nurturing our body, mind, and spirit often falls by the wayside. We push ourselves to the breaking point striving for unattainable standards of perfection until we are left exhausted, anxious, and depleted. But it doesn't have to be this way. Small, intentional daily practices of self-care can profoundly improve our health, outlook, and quality of life.

I learned these lessons the hard way. As a young professional climbing the corporate ladder, I worked tirelessly to succeed. I started each day before sunrise, gulped coffee to stay alert, skipped lunch to attend meetings, stayed late to finish projects, and passed out from stress and exhaustion each night. I was completely burned out but afraid to slow down. My mind and body suffered. I struggled with headaches, insomnia, irritability, and a constant feeling of being overwhelmed. My relationships and health declined. I wasn't living, just surviving each day.

Finally, I realized I desperately needed change before reaching total collapse. I took a step back to reflect on what truly mattered—my well-being and happiness. I wanted to craft a lifestyle that nourished me holistically. So I made self-care a top priority, adopting daily practices to relax and restore myself. As I learned techniques like breath work, home-cooked meals, yoga stretches, and natural beauty remedies, I felt more centered, energetic, and empowered. I left my stressful job and pursued work as a wellness coach helping other women care for themselves. Discovering this passion gave my life meaning. Now I want to share these self-care secrets with you. Like many women, you may resist self-care, thinking it's vain, selfish, or impossible with your busy schedule. But the truth is we can't properly care for others unless we first care for ourselves. Self-care is the key to being mentally and physically well so you can thrive in all areas. My quick, fuss-free tips are designed to fit into any routine. As you gradually make them daily habits, you'll notice a positive change. Your mind will feel calmer, your body healthier, and your outlook more positive. You'll have the energy to pursue your goals and enjoy quality time with loved ones. Don't wait until you're utterly depleted to start caring for YOU. Begin today with small steps for big rewards.

In Natural Wellness Tips for Women, we'll explore holistic self-care in four key areas:

Managing Stress

Today's nonstop, fast-paced world leaves many of us frazzled. We juggle countless duties at home and work while constantly connected to technology in a state of overload. It's a recipe for burnout. Now more than ever, practicing stress relief and relaxation is essential. Science confirms activities like breath work, meditation, yoga, journaling, and time in nature provide powerful mind-body benefits. Just 10-15 minutes per day can rewire your nervous system, lower cortisol, ease anxiety, and prevent stress-related illness. Yet we often skip these practices, wrongly thinking of them as indulgences. I'll share my favorite methods for fitting self-care into even the busiest schedule. You'll learn quick stress relief techniques along with lifestyle changes for more lasting tranquility. With a calm, centered outlook, you'll feel better equipped to thrive amidst daily pressures.

Healthy, Homemade Meals

Hippocrates famously advised, "Let food be thy medicine." What we put into our bodies truly shapes our health and mood. Yet chaotic schedules and reliance on convenience foods often lead to poor diets. Refined carbs, sugar, packaged snacks, and takeout provide little nourishment and leave us depleted. Preparing simple, nutritious home-cooked meals doesn't need to be complicated or time-consuming.It's one of the most loving things we can do for ourselves. I'll provide my go-to recipes for making wholesome breakfasts, lunches, dinners, and snacks you can feel good about. Tips for meal planning, stocking your pantry, batch cooking on weekends and more will take the guesswork out of quick, nutritious eating. Daily nourishing your body with fresh foods supports natural energy, weight management, and overall vitality.

Natural Beauty and Grooming

Good health radiates from within, glowing through vibrant skin, bright eyes, and thick, shiny hair. Yet we often assault our bodies with harsh chemicals in beauty and personal care products. Opting for non-toxic products with wholesome, natural ingredients is an important wellness strategy. Even better, you can easily make many treatments yourself using items from your kitchen! Not only is this more affordable, DIY beauty remedies allow you to customize products to your needs. I'll share my top recipes and tips for homemade skincare, haircare, bath products, and makeup. You'll also learn how developing a signature style that fits your body, personality, and values boosts confidence. When you feel beautiful inside and out, it improves self-esteem and positive body image.

Overall Wellbeing

Caring for health holistically also involves supporting women's wellness needs throughout the lifespan. Getting quality sleep, regular medical screenings, social connections, and emotional support all contribute to optimal well-being. I'll provide tips to help you thrive physically and mentally during life's transitions. You'll learn how setting reasonable goals, reframing thoughts, practicing self-compassion, and celebrating progress can build resilience. Most importantly, remember that wellness is a journey, not a destination. Don't seek perfection, just gradually build healthier habits. Be patient and kind to yourself along the way.

It's my sincerest wish that the guidance in this book helps you slow down and savor the joy of caring for your whole self: body, mind, and spirit. Don't view self-care as a chore or luxury—it's an act of deep self-love. You deserve to feel relaxed, nourished, content, and empowered from the inside out. Are you ready to begin your natural wellness journey? Let's get started!

Chapter 1

Stress Management Techniques for Daily Tranquility

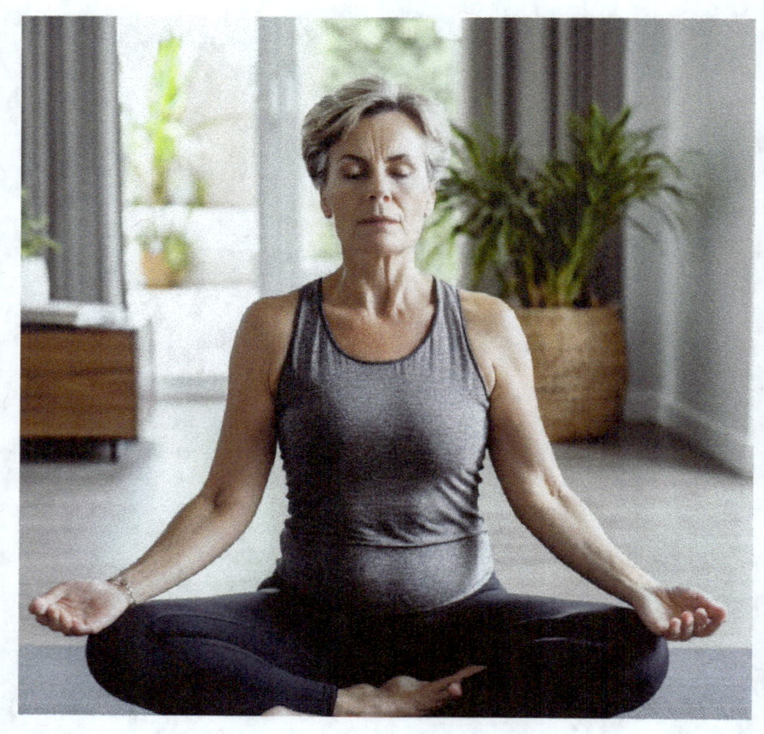

Welcome dear readers join me as we

embark on a wellness journey together! Here, we'll explore ways to manage stress and anxious thoughts through relaxation techniques, mindset shifts, and lifestyle changes. With some simple yet strategic self-care, you can find oases of calm amidst the rush of daily responsibilities.

I know firsthand how overwhelming modern life can feel. Early in my career, I constantly felt frazzled, tense, and on edge. I'd snap at loved ones over minor annoyances and lay awake consumed by worry over work. My neck and shoulders ached from hunching over a computer and my stomach was in knots. Headaches and fatigue left me completely depleted.

This state of constant stress took a real toll on my health and relationships. But I felt pressure to power through. I wrongly saw self-care practices like breaks, boundaries, and relaxation as "luxuries" I didn't have time for.

It wasn't until I ended up at the doctor for stress-related illness that I realized the importance of slowing down. I began researching and testing various stress relief techniques until I created a routine that worked for me. The experts were right—just 10-15 minutes of self-care every day eases anxiety substantially! Over time, activities like breath work, meditation, and yoga became second nature. My frazzled nervous system regained balance through the power of the parasympathetic "rest and digest" response. When stress hits now, I tackle it mindfully rather than spiraling. But I also realized no quick-fix solution can "cure" a stressed life. Setting boundaries, saying no, streamlining obligations, and letting go of perfectionism were essential for lasting calm. I'd wrongly believed relaxing was impossible for a busy career woman. Now I know self-care is about working smarter, not harder. By caring for my needs first, I become better at caring for others without burnout. I have more energy, patience, and joy.

In this chapter, we'll cover:

-How stress affects the body and mind -The benefits of relaxation
-Breathing techniques to try anywhere

-Yoga for beginners

-Meditation and mindfulness demystified

-Aromatherapy and home spa relaxation
-Reframing thoughts through journaling
-Lifestyle changes for ongoing tranquility

Understanding Stress

Let's first define what stress is, beyond a vague feeling of being overwhelmed. At its essence, stress is the body's response to perceived threats and changes. Our ancient ancestors experienced stress when facing life-threatening dangers like predators or enemies. They either quickly fought the threat or took flight to stay alive. We still experience this fight-or-flight response today, but our threats are often emotional like work pressures, financial anxiety, relationship conflicts, or simple daily hassles. When the thinking brain perceives a threat, it signals the nervous system to release hormones like cortisol and adrenaline. Heart rate increases, muscles tense and senses become hyper-alert to deal with the danger.

But chronic triggers leave us in a constant state of physiological stress response that takes a real toll. Tense muscles cause back and neck pain. High blood pressure and increased inflammation raise the risk of heart disease, diabetes, and obesity. Immunity is lowered, making us prone to illness. These physical effects also impact mood, leading to irritability, lack of motivation, and depression. Simply put, stress makes our minds and bodies suffer. Here's the good news: We have the power to reverse the damage through relaxation! Deep breathing, yoga, meditation, and other calming practices re-engage the parasympathetic nervous system. This counteracts fight-or-flight hormones, slowing heart rate, relaxing muscles, lowering blood pressure, and restoring equilibrium. Over time, regular relaxation strengthens the parasympathetic response, making us more resilient to stress. Just 10-15 minutes daily provides profound benefits, both physical and mental. Now let's explore some easy yet effective techniques.

The Healing Benefits of Relaxation

While stress narrows focus to enable immediate survival, relaxation opens awareness and restores inner balance. As Harvard cardiologist Dr. Herbert Benson discovered in his pioneering work, inducing the relaxation response not only alleviates the negative effects of stress — it also boosts immunity, energy, and whole-body health. Some benefits include:

- Lower blood pressure and cortisol

- Slowed heart rate and respiration

- Release of mood-boosting neurotransmitters like serotonin
- Reduced inflammation and pain
- Improved digestion and metabolism
- Enhanced immunity and cardiovascular function
- Increased focus, motivation, and recall memory
- Reduced anxiety, anger and depression
- Improved sleep quality and brain health
- Heightened self-awareness and emotional intelligence Relaxation provides a respite from constant doing to simply be fully present.

Even brief practices deliver myriad benefits for both body and mind. Just remember that relaxation is a skill requiring practice – it may feel

> I'm centered, grounded and at peace.
>
> I gracefully let go of what I cannot control.
>
> I welcome tranquility into my mind, body and spirit.
>
> I am patient and gentle with myself and others.
>
> I lovingly nurture my mind, body and spirit today

uncomfortable at first. Be patient with yourself as you cultivate daily rest periods through these techniques.

Affirmation

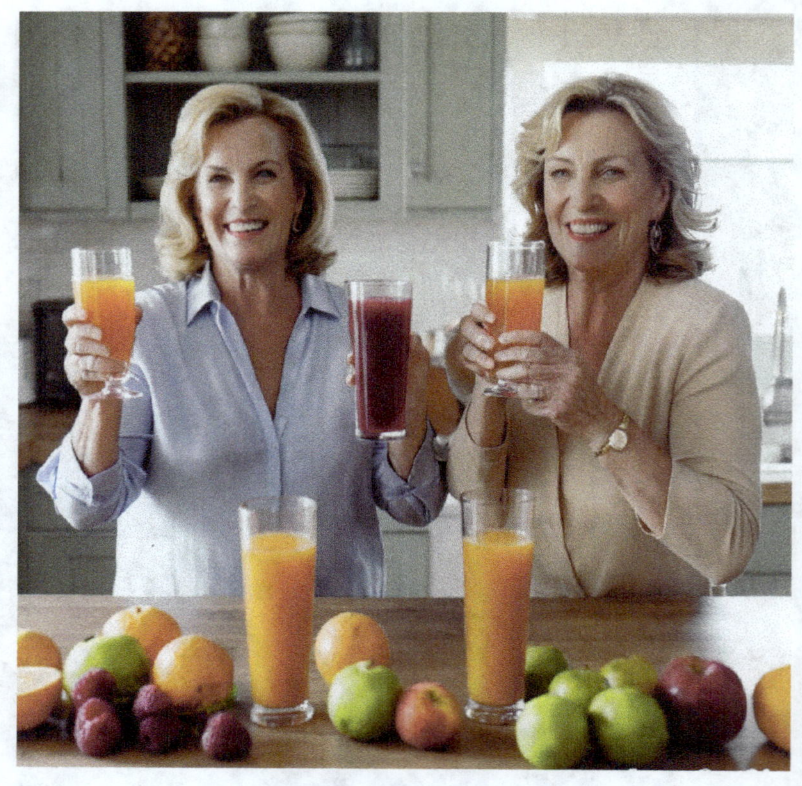

Deep Belly Breathing Anywhere

My busy schedule doesn't always allow an hour for yoga or a bath. When I just need a quick hit of tranquility, I rely on deep breathing. This convenient practice can be done anywhere, anytime!

Breath work taps into our innate relaxation response. It soothes the nervous system by activating the valgus nerve, which connects the brain to major organs. Focusing on breath shifts the brain from stress mode to present-moment awareness. As thoughts wander, gently return focus to each inhale and exhale.

Here's a simple deep breathing exercise:

1. Sit or stand tall with relaxed, bent knees. Close your eyes if possible.
2. Place one hand on your chest, and the other on your belly.

3. Inhale slowly and deeply through your nose, feeling air expand your belly.

4. Exhale just as slowly through pursed lips, pressing out all air as your belly contracts.

5. Repeat for 5-10 cycles, focusing only on smooth inhales and complete exhales.

Remember to breathe from your diaphragm, not shallow chest breaths.

Fill your belly like a balloon on each inhale. Slow, complete exhales help relax muscles and calm the nervous system. Just a few minutes can lower cortisol and clear your mind.

Once you've mastered the basic technique, you can practice anytime during stressful moments: while stuck in traffic, or when frustrated with your toddler during a difficult conversation. Over time, mindful breathing first thing in the morning and last thing at night changes automatic stress reactions into relaxation.

Yoga Stretches for Beginners

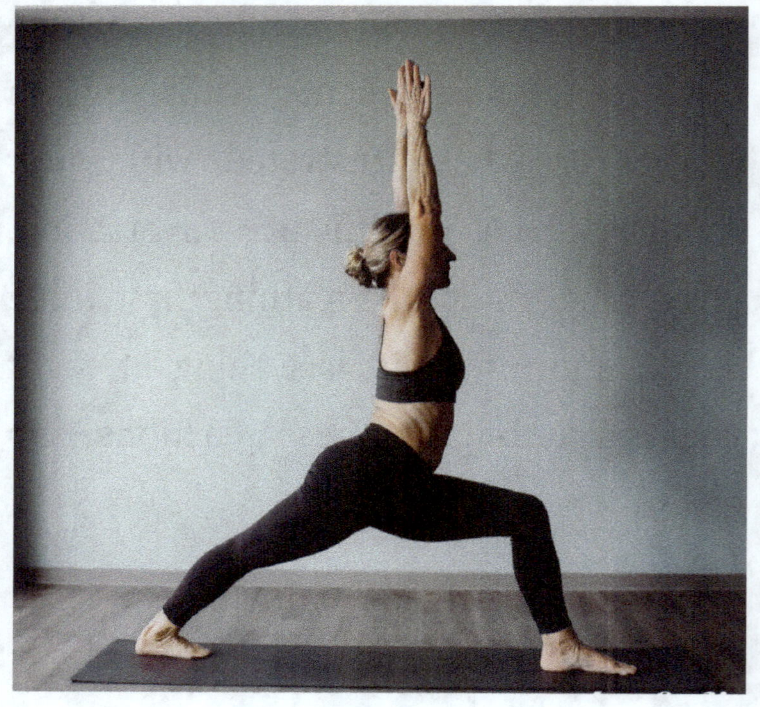

The term "yoga" often brings to mind advanced poses and spiritual mysticism. But yoga is quite simply the practice of union between mind and body. The physical poses serve to support mindfulness, flexibility, and strength.

Don't be intimidated if you're a beginner or "inflexible." There are yoga techniques suitable for all levels. The most important thing is to focus on how each movement makes your body feel without judgment.

Yoga's benefits are proven by science: improved heart health, immunity, emotional regulation, sleep quality and cognitive functions. Moving through postures with full awareness brings us into the present moment. Holding poses challenges the mind to release negative thoughts and embrace stillness. Linking movement to breath helps this process. As you inhale and exhale smoothly, relaxation arises naturally. Starting with just 10-15 minutes whenever you can makes yoga benefits accessible. There are options for all ability levels.

Here are two foundational starter poses:

- Child's Pose –

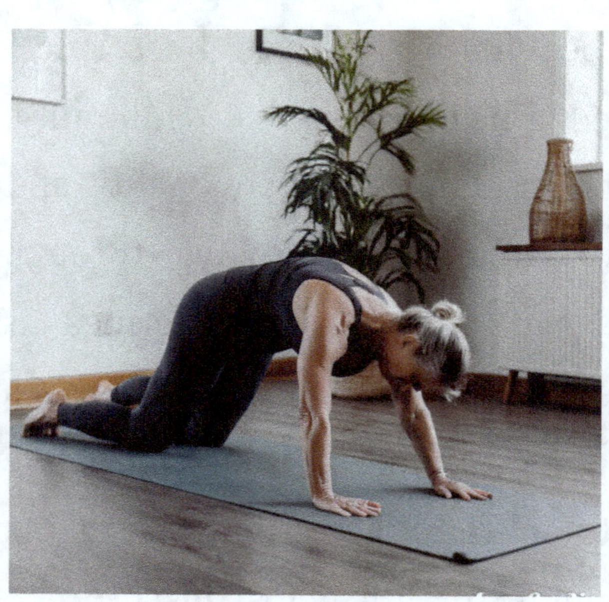

Kneel with toes together and knees hip-width apart. Exhale as you sink your hips toward your feet, arms extended forward. This gently stretches the hips, thighs, and spine. Hold for 5 deep breaths.

- Legs Up the Wall -

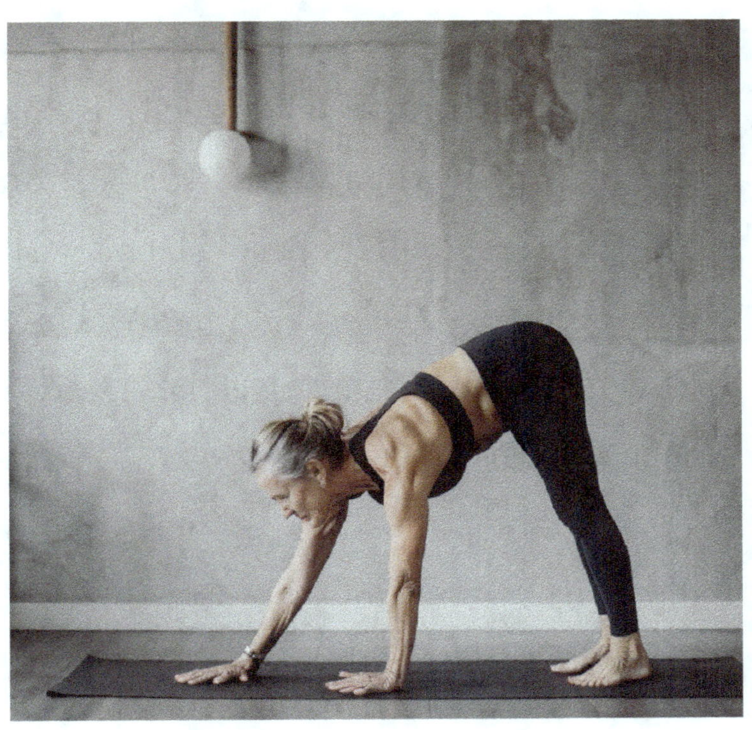

Lie on your back with legs resting against a wall, hips and knees bent at 90 degrees. Arms rest at your sides, palms facing up. Breathe deeply for 5-10 minutes focusing on sensations of gentle stretch.

I recommend taking beginner yoga classes if possible. The instructor can help you find proper alignment. But a great option is Yoga With Adriene on **YouTube** — she offers free videos for all levels. Find what feels right for your body as it is today. Relax into stretches instead of aggressively "pushing through." Yoga isn't about perfection - it's about mind-body awareness.

Meditation Made Simple The word meditation often brings to mind monks sitting silently for hours, completely emptying the mind. As a busy working mom, I used to think I could never meditate successfully. But in truth, meditation means simply focusing your attention on the present moment without judgment. Start with short, gentle sessions, and don't get frustrated by wandering thoughts. Over time and practice, you can build up to longer meditations with less mind chatter.

A simple way to start is mindful breathing:

- Sit comfortably with eyes closed and back straight but relaxed. Set a timer for 2-5 minutes.
- Bring all your attention to inhaling and exhaling slowly and deeply.
- When thoughts arise, notice them and then gently return focus to breath.
- Don't judge yourself for wandering - just keep returning to the breath.

Once you've practiced mindful breathing for a few weeks, try "body scans." Lie down, close your eyes, and slowly notice any sensations in each body part from head to toe. Don't analyze sensations, just acknowledge them. This builds greater mind-body awareness.

You can meditate at any time with your eyes open or closed. While washing dishes, walking, brushing your teeth, or waiting in line, come back to your breath or bodily sensations again and again.

Over time, you may work up to 20-30 minute seated sessions. But any practice helps calm and center your mind.

Aromatherapy and Home Spa Self-Care

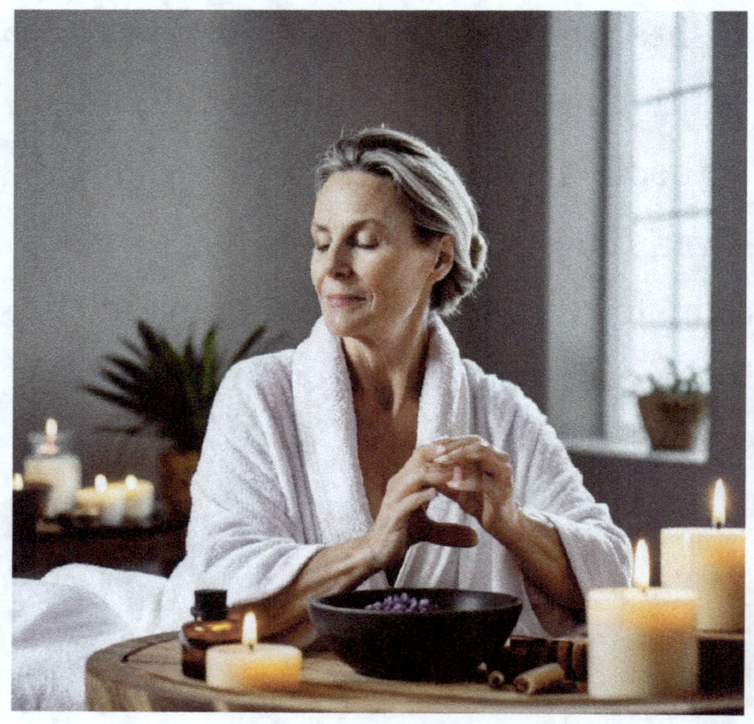

Who doesn't enjoy relaxing at a spa? There's something deeply restorative about soothing services like massages, saunas, and aromatherapy treatments.

But the time and expense of regular spa visits just aren't realistic for most of us. Luckily, you can recreate that tranquil ambiance right at home with a few self-care essentials. Set aside an hour each week for your own mini spa experience and feel stress melt away!
Here are some of my at-home spa tips:

- Soak in a hot Epsom salt bath by candlelight with essential oils lavender promotes calm and eucalyptus opens airways
- Give yourself a facial massage with almond or coconut oil to hydrate skin

- Brew tea with fresh herbs like chamomile, peppermint or lemon balm

- Mix essential oils like bergamot, clary sage or frankincense into an oil burner or diffuser

- Make a hydrating and soothing hair mask with avocado, honey and olive oil

- Give yourself a neck and shoulder massage with calming essential oils

- Listen to spa relaxation music, nature sounds or guided meditation during treatments

The key is creating an ambiance free of other distractions. Switch off phones and screens. Light candles, play soft music and savor these moments focusing only on your senses. The simple ritual shifts awareness from busy thoughts to simply being present and caring for yourself. Journaling for Emotional Wellbeing

Writing about emotions, challenges, and goals can positively impact both mental and physical health. Journaling allows you to reflect, gain clarity and release feelings productively. Putting experiences into words activates different neural pathways than simply ruminating on events. It facilitates learning, insight, and integrating experiences into your self-narrative. Research shows journaling reduces stress, anxiety and depression while improving immune function. It's an excellent tool for understanding thought patterns, beliefs and emotional triggers. With hectic schedules, making time to journal may feel impossible. But just 5-10 minutes of stream-of-consciousness writing whenever you can provides benefits. There's no need for perfect grammar or editing. Simply get thoughts and emotions out of your head. Regular journaling helps release negativity, cultivate gratitude, solve problems and achieve goals.

Here are journaling tips for beginners:

- Write first thing in the morning or before bed when your mind is calm and open.

- Set a timer for 5-10 minutes and keep writing without stopping.
- Start with "I am feeling..." or

  "Today I'm grateful for..."

- Elaborate on emotions, experiences, challenges and goals.
- Close entries feeling peaceful, not dwelling on problems.
- Reread entries over time to gain perspective on growth.

Journaling can be cathartic during times of stress or transition. It also serves to clarify goals, priorities and next steps when feeling stuck. Over time, reflecting on entries helps reinforce positive thought patterns and behaviors supporting wellness.

Crafting a Lifestyle of Calm

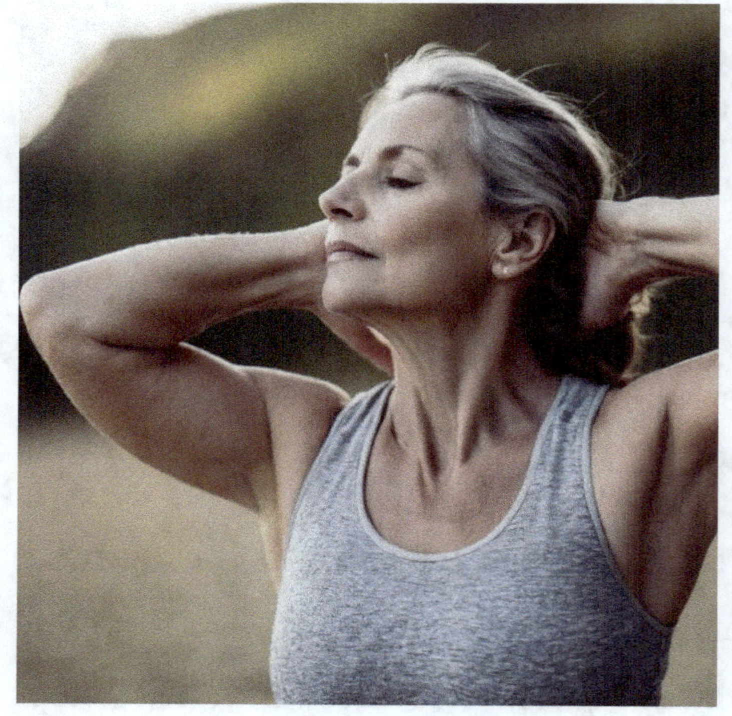

Quick stress relief practices help tremendously in the moment. But if demanding obligations and perfectionism constantly keep your nervous system in overdrive, you'll struggle to find lasting peace. Take time to reflect on changes that could help your lifestyle align better with your values and well-being needs. Here are some areas to consider:

Boundaries/Saying No - Does your schedule fit reasonable time for work, relationships, self-care, fun, and rest? Do you agree to unnecessary obligations from a desire to people, please? Practice saying no to nonessential duties. Protect your energy.

Simplifying/Streamlining - Do you spend time on tasks that don't ultimately matter that much? Delegate or eliminate activities that don't align with your priorities. Practice the 80/20 rule of efficiency.

Technology/Social Media - Do you find yourself endlessly scrolling and reacting instead of meaningfully engaging? Set limits on screen time to be fully present with loved ones. Unplug completely at least one day per week.

Perfectionism - Are you putting excessive pressure on yourself? Perfection isn't possible or healthy. Focus on consistent progress, not outcomes. Give yourself grace.

Letting Go of Worry - Are you ruminating over things outside your control? Redirect worries into positive action when possible. Release the rest through coping strategies.

There are no quick fixes to instantly transform a stressed life. But over time, choosing what matters and building in daily self-care empowers you to feel balanced and peaceful. Be patient with the process.

In closing, I hope you feel ready to start reducing stress through relaxation techniques and thoughtful lifestyle choices. Consistent practice is key, even when life feels too chaotic. Honor your **well-being** – you are worth it. Let go of perfectionism and take things one small step at a time. By caring for your mind and body first, you'll have energy left over to care for others. You've got this! Now go relax. **Some stress Management tips**

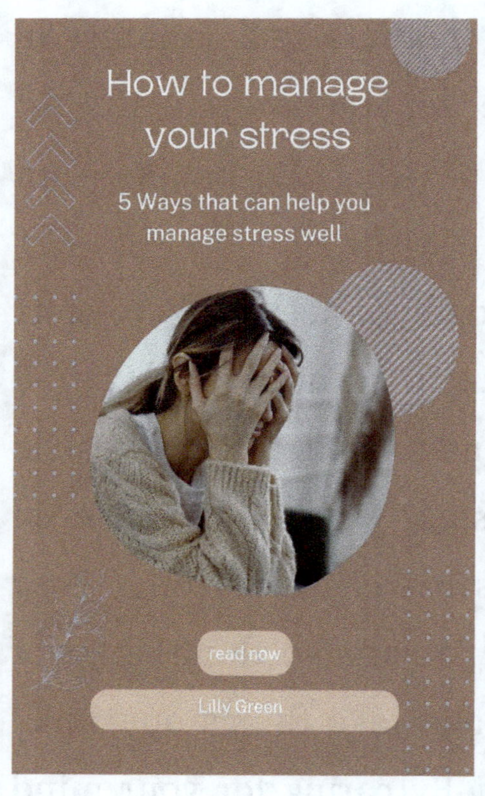

Take breaks from watching, reading, or listening to news stories,

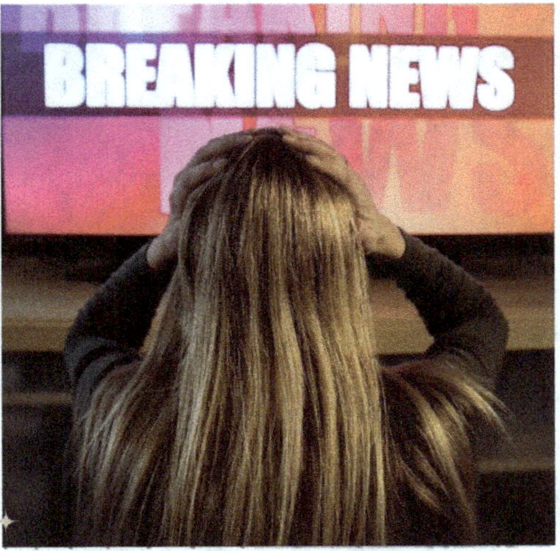

including those on social media. It's good to be informed but hearing about the traumatic event constantly can be upsetting. Consider limiting news to just a couple of times a day and disconnecting from phone, tv, and computer screens for a while

Lilly Green

Take care of your body

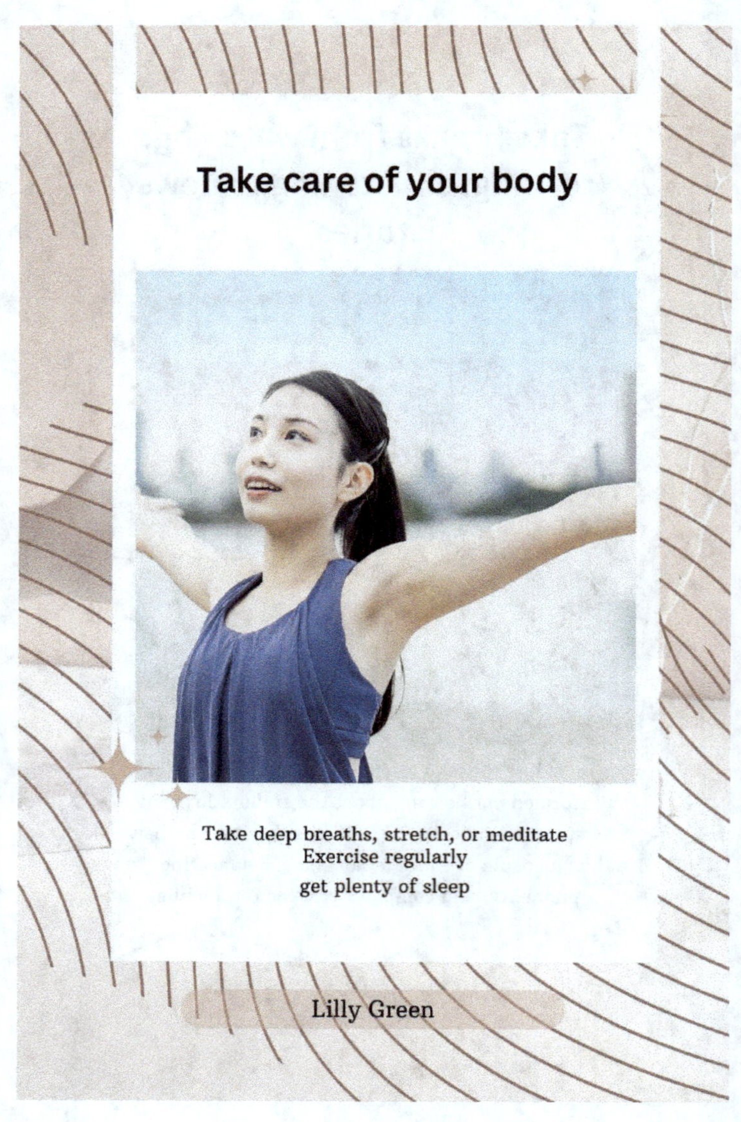

Take deep breaths, stretch, or meditate
Exercise regularly

get plenty of sleep

Lilly Green

Avoid drugs and alcohol

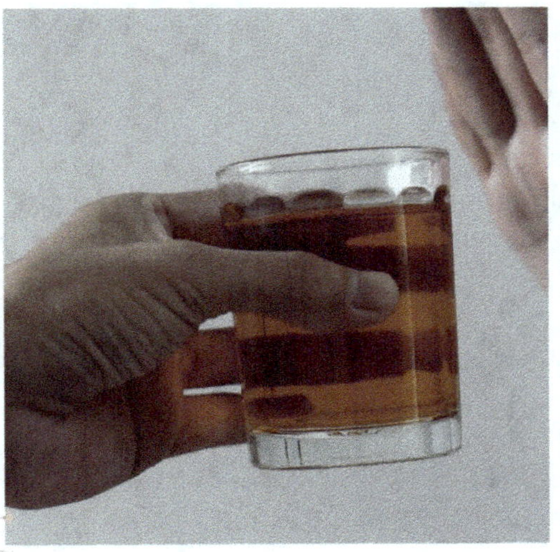

These may seem to help, but they can create additional problems and increase the stress you are already feeling.

Lilly Green

Take care of yourself

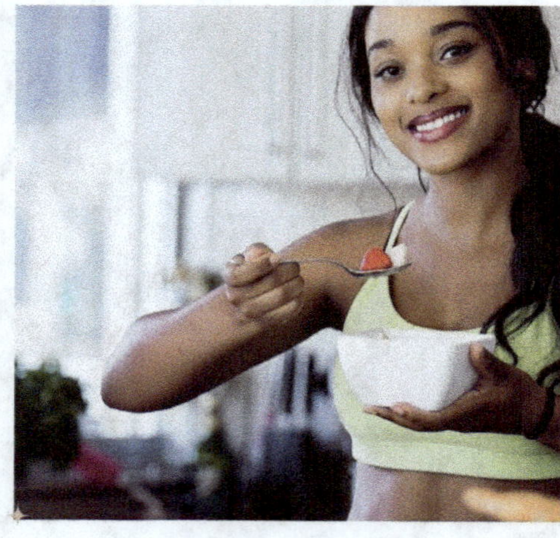

Eat healthy, exercise, get plenty of sleep, and give yourself a break if you feel stressed out.

Lilly Green

Connect with your community- or faith-based organizations.

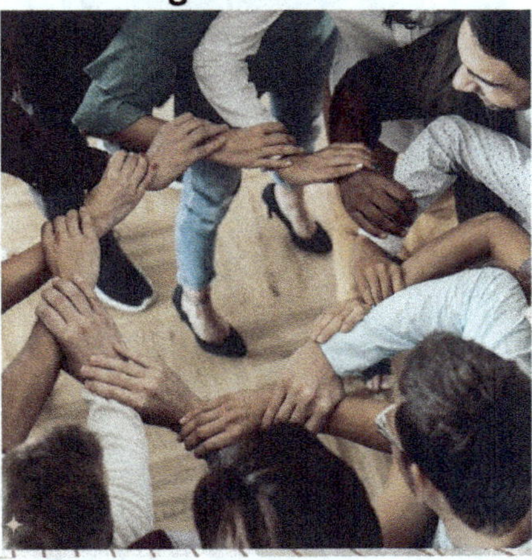

Talking with someone you trust can help you make sense out of your experience. Or a faith based community, If you are not sure where to turn, call your local crisis intervention center or a national hotline.

Lilly Green

Chapter 2

Healthy, Homemade Meals to Nourish Body and Mind

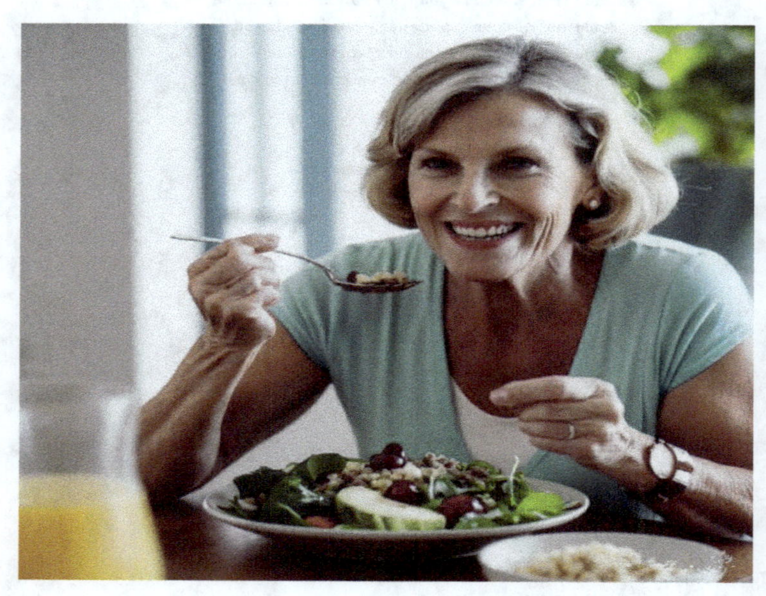

Welcome to another Chapter of our wellness journey focusing on the healing power of homemade, nutritious food! Like many people today, I once relied on rushed, convenient meals that left me undernourished. I'd grab an egg sandwich on the way to work, nibble on vending machine snacks between meetings, order takeout for dinner, and wonder why I felt utterly depleted. It wasn't until illness forced me to rethink my diet that I realized food's profound impact on health.

What we regularly put into our bodies becomes the very building blocks of our cells, tissues, organs, and energy levels.

When we opt for overly processed, sugary, chemical-laden convenience foods, we deny our bodies essential vitamins, minerals, antioxidants, and more. This leads to inflammation, weight gain, disease risks, and lackluster moods. Many chronic health conditions are aggravated or even caused by nutritional deficiencies.

But when we nourish ourselves with real, fresh, home-cooked foods, it's like medicine from within. Vibrant salads, savory beans, antioxidant-rich fruits, healthy fats, herbs, spices and more provide our cells with the tools they need to function optimally. Mealtime becomes an opportunity to love ourselves through wholesome ingredients prepared with care.

In this chapter, we'll explore:

- How diet impacts mental and physical health
- Strategies for easier home cooking
- Ingredients for a well-stocked kitchen
- Nourishing but fast breakfast ideas
- Packable lunches and snacks
- Simple weeknight dinner recipes
- Satisfying one-dish meals
- Naturally sweetened desserts

Let's get started cooking up wellness! This chapter will equip you with tips and simple recipes to get delicious, nutritious meals on the table every day.

Diet and Wellness

There's no doubt you've heard the phrase "You are what you eat." But have you truly considered its powerful truth? The foods making up your daily diet directly impact every function of your body and mind. A poor diet jeopardizes health, while a nutrient-rich diet protects it.

Diet affects energy levels, weight, gastrointestinal function, immune strength, hormonal balance, heart health, inflammation, disease risks, and even mental health. For example, a diet high in processed carbs and sugary foods leads to crashes and fatigue as blood sugar spikes and plummets. Excess saturated fat intake correlates to heart disease, obesity, and diabetes risk. Nutrient deficiencies brought on by a highly restricted diet can cause anemia, osteoporosis, migraines, and more.

On the flip side, getting a rainbow of anti-inflammatory phytonutrients from vegetables lowers inflammation tied to just about every chronic illness. Lean proteins provide essential amino acids to build and repair tissue. Whole grains offer sustained energy and digestion-friendly fiber. Good fats like olive oil, avocados, and oily fish support heart health, hormones, and brain function.

Truly, food can be thy medicine – protecting against disease and dysfunction. A diet of mostly whole, minimally processed foods nourishes us from a cellular level, empowering vibrant well-being. Making simple, nutritious choices each day prevents depletion and conditions the body to thrive. With some effortless strategies like meal planning, batch cooking, and keeping a stocked pantry, it's easy to get wholesome home-cooked meals on the table without becoming a full-time chef!

Let's explore some kitchen tips...

Strategies for Easier Home Cooking

Preparing satisfying meals from scratch each day may sound daunting, but it doesn't have to be. With a bit of planning and practice, nutritious home cooking becomes second nature. You'll get a feel for throwing together simple yet nourishing meals that fit your preferences and schedule.

Here are my top tips for quick, easy home cooking:

- Review recipe ideas and plan out weekly meals – include one-dish

meals, slow cooker, and 30-minute
options.

- Prep ingredients or entire recipes in
  advance on less busy days.
- Stock up on hearty basics like whole
  grains, beans, veggies, eggs, and
  lean proteins.
- Freeze pre-portioned meals in
  individual containers to simply
  reheat on busy nights.
- Enlist help from family to chop
  vegetables, make salads, etc.
- Double recipes and use leftovers for
  lunches or a second meal later in
  the week.

- Incorporate seasonal produce to cut down on chopping with faster roasting or sautéing.

Use shortcuts like pre-chopped veggies and rotisserie chicken when you need them.

Try new gadgets like an air fryer, instant pot, salad spinner, or veggie chopper.

Simplify with a one-sheet pan or slow cooker meals needing little hands-on time.

Make extra on less busy days to stock your freezer with healthy convenience meals.

With practice, you'll discover which approaches fit your lifestyle best. The key is finding harmony between wholesome eating and a realistic schedule. Now let's get you set up with a stellar kitchen!

Stocking an Optimal Kitchen Having the right foods on hand makes throwing together a home-cooked meal infinitely easier. A well-stocked pantry and fridge should contain most raw ingredients you need for balanced meals and snacks on a regular basis. Shop weekly and restock staples before running out. Here's an overview of items to keep on hand:

Pantry:

- Whole grains (brown rice, oats, quinoa, whole-wheat pasta)
- Canned fish (salmon, sardines)
- Beans and lentils
- Seeds and nuts

- Oils (olive, avocado, sesame, coconut)

- Vinegars (balsamic, apple cider)

- Herbs, spices, stocks, sauces

- Canned or jarred vegetables

- Nut butters

Fridge:

- Eggs

- Fresh or frozen fruits/veggies

- Yogurt, cottage cheese

- Hummus, fresh salsa

- Leftover cooked grains and proteins

- Condiments like mustard, hot sauce

  Freezer:

- Frozen fruits and vegetables

- Breads or pitas

- Meat and fish.

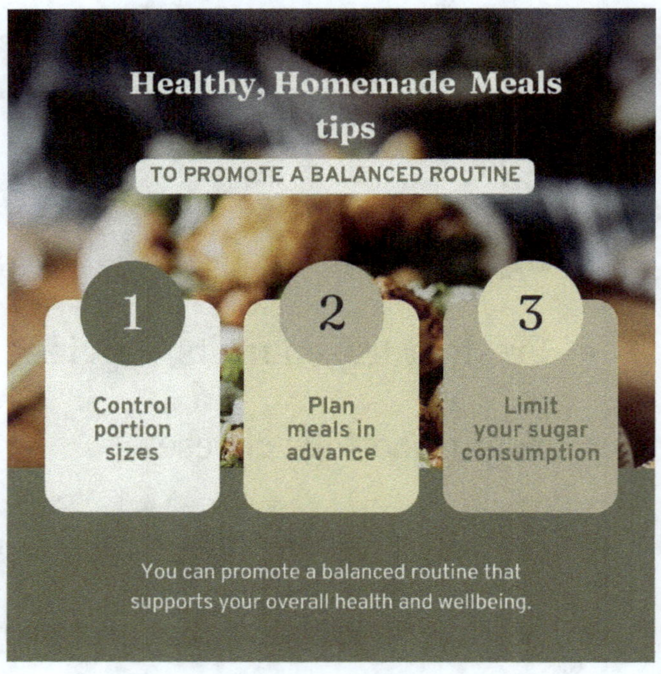

Frozen meals and leftovers Having staple ingredients on hand makes preparing healthy meals so much simpler. You can easily whip up omelets, grain bowls, salads, sandwiches, sheet pan meals and more. Let's get cooking!

Nourishing Breakfasts

Many of us skip breakfast or opt for a sugary pastry on-the-go. But taking a few minutes to nourish your body first thing empowers your best day. A protein-rich breakfast provides satiety, sustained energy and mental clarity instead of a mid-morning crash. Here are nourishing breakfasts you can make quickly:

Veggie Egg Muffins – Whisk eggs with milk or water. Add any veggies and bake in a muffin tin. Enjoy hot or cold weather.

- Yogurt Bowl – Top Greek yogurt with fruit, nuts, chia seeds and a drizzle of honey.

- Peanut Butter & Banana Toast – Spread nut butter and banana slices on whole grain bread.

- Protein Smoothie – Blend milk or a milk alternative with protein

- powder, fruit, spinach, nut butter or oats.

- Avocado Toast – Mash avocado onto whole grain toast and top with an egg, hot sauce, herbs, etc. Overnight Oats – Mix oats with milk and preferred toppings, then refrigerate overnight.
- Breakfast Burrito – Scramble eggs and veggies, wrap in a whole grain tortilla with salsa or hot sauce.

With a little prep, you can have pre-portioned egg muffins, smoothie packs and overnight oats ready to grab and go! Having quick, satisfying options makes mornings smoother.

Simple Lunches and Snacks Come mid-day, avoid vending machine junk food that leaves you hungrier an hour later. Pack lunches with a balance of fiber, protein and healthy fats for sustained energy and focus. For effortless snacks, keep washed fruits and veggies, nuts, cottage cheese, yogurt and hummus stocked. Here are nourishing lunch ideas to pack up:

Veggie Rice Bowl – Cooked grains with sauteed veggies, greens, beans, tofu, avocado and dressing

Mason Jar Salad – Layer salad ingredients like greens, chickpeas, nuts, dressing in a jar for lunch-on-the-go.

Veggie Wrap/Sandwich – Hummus, cucumber, peppers, spinach and sprouts wrapped in a tortilla or whole grain bread.

Cottage Cheese and Fruit – Sprinkle flax or pumpkin seeds over cottage cheese with berries, melon or apples

Protein & Apple – Nut butter or portable string cheese paired with apple slices.

Energy Bites – Make no-bake bites with oats, nuts, dried fruit, nut butter, etc. Grab a few for snack time.

- **Trail Mix** – Toss together nuts, seeds, coconut flakes, dried fruit in a baggie for on-the-go munching. Simple swaps like opting for yogurt or fruit instead of doughnuts, trail mix not chips, and water over soda lets you snack smarter at the office, at home or on the run. You'll stay full and focused without energy crashes.

30-Minute Weeknight Dinners

Weeknight meals need to be fast but nourishing. With whole food ingredients and minimal prep, you can get a complete meal on the table in 30 minutes or less. The key is sticking to simple recipes with fresh produce, whole grains, lean proteins and healthy fats. Here are some favorite quick dinner recipes:

- Sheet Pan Salmon & Veggies – Place wild salmon filets and chopped veggies tossed in olive oil on a rimmed baking sheet. Bake at 400F for 15-20 minutes.
- Turkey Lettuce Wraps – Quickly sauté ground turkey or crumble tempeh, adding salsa, beans, etc. Serve in butter lettuce leaves.

- Veggie & Tofu Stir Fry – Slice veggies and lightly marinate tofu while cooking brown rice. Then stir fry everything in a skillet with your favorite sauce.

- Fajita Bowls – Sauté onions, peppers and spices, serve over rice and beans. Top with avocado and Greek yogurt.

- Greens & Grain Bowl – Cook quinoa and sautéed greens like kale or spinach. Top with roasted squash, chickpeas, hemp hearts, dressing.

- Chicken & Sweet Potato Soup – Sauté aromatics, add broth, cream and diced sweet potato. Simmer until tender and add cooked chicken.

With the right tools like a sharp knife, meal planning and prep, you can make fast, satisfying dinners any night of the week. Set a fun family table and relax together over nourishing fare.

Simple One-Dish Wonders

Using a slow cooker, instant pot or oven, you can create divine hands-off dishes with your pantry staples. These require minimal chopping or stove time - just dump ingredients in and let the appliance do the work! Here are effortless one-dish recipes:

- Chili – Brown ground turkey or crumble tempeh, add canned tomatoes, beans, seasonings and

stock. Simmer for 20-30 minutes
for a hearty, protein-rich meal.
Serve over rice or baked potatoes.

- Rice & Bean Bowls – Combine rice,

  canned beans, garlic, veggies, spices
  and broth. Cook in a rice cooker or
  Instant Pot. Top with avocado, salsa
  and Greek yogurt.

- Lentil Soup – Sauté aromatics, add
  lentils and broth spiced with cumin,
  coriander and turmeric. Cook until
  lentils are tender. Blend for
  smoothness as desired.

- Chicken Casserole – Season chicken
  breasts or thighs with herbs, layer
  in a baking dish with milk, broth,
  veggies and whole grain noodles.

Cover and bake at 375 F for 45 minutes to 1 hour.

- Overnight Steel Cut Oats – Combine oats, chia seeds, nuts and dried fruit in a slow cooker. Add milk, cinnamon and vanilla. Cook on low overnight. Wake up to perfect oatmeal!

- Eggplant Parmesan – Layer sliced eggplant, tomato sauce and cheese in a baking dish. Cover and bake for 40 minutes until bubbly. Serve over pasta tossed with pesto.

Letting appliances do the cooking means you can enjoy time with family or relaxing instead of slaving at the stove. Using nutritious pantry staples results in home-cooked goodness with little effort required.

Naturally Sweetened Desserts You can absolutely enjoy sweet treats as part of a healthy diet when you opt for better ingredients. Focus on whole foods over heavily processed items full of refined sugar and additives. Here are some nourishing desserts with just a touch of natural sweetness:

- Greek Yogurt Parfaits – Layer yogurt with fruit, nuts, shredded coconut, cacao nibs, chia seeds, etc. Sweeten with a drizzle of maple syrup or honey if desired.

- Banana "Ice Cream" – Blend frozen bananas into a creamy, ice

cream-like treat. Swirl in nut butter
or cacao powder for added flavor
and nutrition.

- Protein Cookies – Mix oats, nut
  butter, protein powder, coconut and
  dark chocolate chips. Scoop dough
  and bake for 8-10 minutes.

- Strawberry Chia Pudding – Blend
  coconut milk, vanilla extract and
  strawberries. Stir in chia seeds and
  refrigerate to thicken. Top with
  coconut flakes.

- Avocado Chocolate Pudding –
  Blend avocado, cacao powder and
  milk for a decadent chocolate
  pudding. Sweeten with maple syrup
  and top with fruit.

- Coconut Milk Fudge – Mix melted coconut oil with cacao powder, coconut milk and your choice of mix-ins like nuts or dried fruit. Pour into a dish and refrigerate until firm.

Treat yourself to nutritious sweets a few times per week after nourishing meals. You can have your cake and eat it too when opting for better ingredients! In closing, I hope this chapter revealed that home cooking doesn't have to be difficult or time consuming. With a well-stocked kitchen, meal planning and some simple recipes, you can nourish yourself and family with delicious, nutrient-dense foods. When diet supports overall wellness, you'll feel more energized, empowered and resilient in body and mind. Here's to home cooking as an act of true self-care!

Meal Planning Made Simple

Planning out a week's worth of meals in advance can transform your home cooking experience. It reduces the nightly question of "What's for dinner?" and ensures you have ingredients ready for each recipe. You'll gain confidence in the kitchen knowing meals are handled! To plan, first take inventory of what's already in your pantry, fridge and freezer. Then create a shopping list for any missing ingredients. Look at your calendar for the week – which nights allow more time for cooking, which need 30-minute meals? Here are helpful tips:

- Focus on dishes that use common ingredients like eggs, beans, rice, veggies, chicken.
- Double up on ingredients needed for multiple meals like cooked chicken for salads and enchiladas.
- Incorporate leftovers into the plan like extra chili or roasted veggies for quick lunches.
- Include a couple one-dish meals you can make in a slow cooker or sheet pan.

- Balance heavier and lighter meals throughout the week.
- Schedule any prep work like cooking grains and chopping veggies in advance.

Planning around your on-hand staples and schedule prevents wasting ingredients. Prepping ahead saves time when it's crunch time for dinner. Most importantly, a weekly meal plan curbs the temptation for last-minute unhealthy takeout on busy nights!

Grocery Shopping Strategies An organized grocery list based on your meal plan ensures you shop efficiently. But it's easy to get sidetracked once you hit the store aisles. Follow these tips to make quick work of grocery trips:

- Stick to the perimeter first for whole foods like produce, meat, eggs and dairy before venturing to inner aisles.

- Compare prices of generic, store brand vs name brand packaged items. Opt for the most budget-friendly.

- Scan shelves from top to bottom – pricier items are generally placed at eye level.

- Check the unit price when comparing different package sizes. Bigger isn't necessarily better.

- Purchase produce in season when prices tend to be lower.

- Pick up an extra hearty veggie like squash, sweet potatoes or cauliflower to roast for easy side dishes all week.

- Resist impulse buys! Stick to your list, except for a new spice or ingredient you want to try in a planned recipe.

A few organizational habits make shopping efficient and affordable. Cook once, eat multiple times by planning recipes with overlapping ingredients. And freeze any extras to enjoy later!

Meal Prep Tips and Tricks

Who doesn't dream of free time? Make it reality by preparing ingredients or entire recipes on less busy days to enjoy throughout the week. Pre-chopped veggies and batch cooked items are life-changing!

- Roast sheet pans of seasonal veggies to use in multiple dishes like grain bowls, sandwiches, soups and casseroles.

- Cook a double batch of whole grains like brown rice or farro to use in lunches or quick dinners.

- Grill, bake or rotisserie an extra chicken breast. Shred meat for easy additions to tacos, wraps, soups, etc.

- Prep salad ingredients or mason jar ingredients to assemble quickly for weekday lunches.

- Whip up a big batch of energy bites, granola bars or chia pudding to have grab-and-go snacks.

- Mix up flavorful sauces, dressings or spice mixes to add instant flavor to dishes all week.

- Assemble breakfast sandwiches or burritos and individually wrap to freeze. Reheat for fast mornings.

- Portion savory dishes like chili, casseroles and soups into containers to freeze. Enjoy later in the week or month!

A little strategic preparation over the weekends allows you to simply reheat and assemble healthy meals when weekday time is limited. Invest some time now and reap benefits all week long!

Inexpensive Plant-Based Proteins

Meat and fish certainly provide protein, but they aren't the only options. Beans, lentils, nuts and even greens offer a healthful dose of plant-based protein. Center meals around these affordable proteins to cut costs without sacrificing nutrition!

Canned Beans – Protein-packed and budget-friendly! Chickpeas, black or pinto beans are versatile additions to soups, salads, tacos, rice bowls and more. Rinse before using to reduce sodium.

Lentils – These fiber-rich legumes cook faster than beans and blend smoothly for hearty vegetarian soups and stews. Red lentils break down into a texture similar to ground beef. Brown and green lentils hold their shape.

Tofu & Tempeh – Made from soy, both pack a hefty protein punch and absorb flavors easily. Press and marinate or crumble tempeh to use like ground meat. Add baked, seasoned tofu to stir fries, broth soups and noodle bowls.

Nuts & Nut Butters – Stock up on nuts and nut butters like almond or peanut to add protein, healthy fats and flavor to meals and snacks. Try nut-based cream sauces or salad dressings.

Greens – Leafy greens like kale, spinach and arugula contain a few grams of protein per serving. Add handfuls to smoothies, scrambles, pasta dishes, **soups** – anywhere you can hide more veggies!

Flavorful plant proteins help cut meal costs without sacrificing nutrition, variety or taste. Embrace veggies, beans and lentils in place of pricey packaged convenience foods for home cooking on a budget.

Sneaky Ways to Increase Veggies
Boosting your daily vegetable and fruit intake positively impacts almost every aspect of health. But when life gets busy, produce can fall by the wayside. Get clever with these stealthy ideas to work more into meals and snacks:

- Add spinach, zucchini or mushrooms to meatloaf or burgers
- Blend cauliflower into mac and cheese or mashed potatoes
- Mix berries or bananas into overnight oats or smoothies
- Serve veggie-loaded soups like minestrone for dinner with whole grain bread

- Snack on carrots, peppers, edamame and hummus throughout the day
- Sauté onion, bell pepper and baby spinach into eggs or egg scrambles
- Toss extra veggies into pasta sauce, chili, curry and stir fries
- Make "noodles" from zucchini using a spiralizer for quick noodle replacements
- Mix shredded carrots or zucchini into meatballs, energy bites and quick breads
- Freeze extra fruit like berries or bananas to add to yogurt, oatmeal and smoothies

With a sprinkle of creativity, you can incorporate vegetables and fruits into meals in place of other ingredients. Boost nutrition without even realizing it!

Simple Smoothie Boosts

A nutrient dense smoothie makes an ideal quick breakfast or snack. But basic fruit and yogurt blends can become boring fast. Amp up nutrition with mix-ins that also add delicious flavors and textures!

Protein Powder – Whey or plant-based protein powders infuse a protein punch that sustains energy and keeps you full.

Nut or Seed Butter – Nutrient-packed additions like almond or sunflower seed butter make smoothies creamier.

Frozen Veggies – Spinach, kale, cauliflower and even zucchini blend smoothly when frozen. You won't even taste them!

Chia or Hemp Seeds – These tiny superfood seeds add omega-3's, fiber and thickness to your blend.

Oats or Granola – Adding a handful boosts staying power and benefits digestion.

Cacao Nibs or Powder – Add antioxidants and satisfy chocolate cravings with crunchy cacao nibs or sweet powder.

Cinnamon – This anti-inflammatory spice adds a hint of sweetness without any sugar.

Fresh Herbs – Mint, basil, parsley or cilantro impart natural flavor when blended.

With endless combinations, you can create a different health-boosting smoothie every day of the week. They're perfect for breakfasts on the go or afternoon pick-me-ups.

Natural Homemade Electrolyte Drink

Skip the artificial dyes, flavors and sweeteners found in popular sports drinks that can actually hinder hydration.

Making your own electrolyte beverage is easy with just a few natural ingredients. It replenishes the body after exercise or during illness.

Combine the following in a large pitcher or liter bottle of water. Shake or stir to incorporate.

- Sea salt or Himalayan salt – 1/ teaspoon
- Fresh lemon or lime juice – 2 tablespoons
- Maple syrup or raw honey (optional)

– 1 tablespoon • Fresh mint leaves (optional)

For added electrolytes and minerals:

- Coconut water – 1 cup

- Magnesium powder – 1 teaspoon

  Hydrate naturally with this refreshingly flavored drink. The simple ingredients provide an optimal balance of sodium, glucose, potassium, magnesium and more to recharge your body's cells.

Anytime Snacks for Energy

It's normal for energy and mood to fluctuate throughout the day. Be prepared with healthy snacks to give yourself an instant boost when you hit a slump. Combining protein, fiber and healthy fats sustains energy for hours. Here are go-to picks for any time:

- Apple or celery sticks with nut or seed butter
- Greek yogurt topped with nuts and cinnamon
- Cottage cheese and fruit
- Veggies and hummus
- Hard Boiled egg and whole grain crackers
- Energy bites made with oats, nuts, dried fruit
- Whole grain toast with nut butter and banana
- Trail mix with nuts, seeds, dried fruit Keep effortless snacks stocked at home, work and on-the-go. You'll   sidestep impulse vending

machine purchases and arrive at meals feeling truly hungry, not ravenous. Quick bites of wholesome food keep you energized all day.

Whew, we covered so much helpful territory to simplify home cooking! What tips are you most excited to try for nourishing, delicious meals? Remember, each dish is an opportunity to care for yourself with the gift of health-giving foods. Here's to joyful, stress-free time together in the kitchen and around the table!

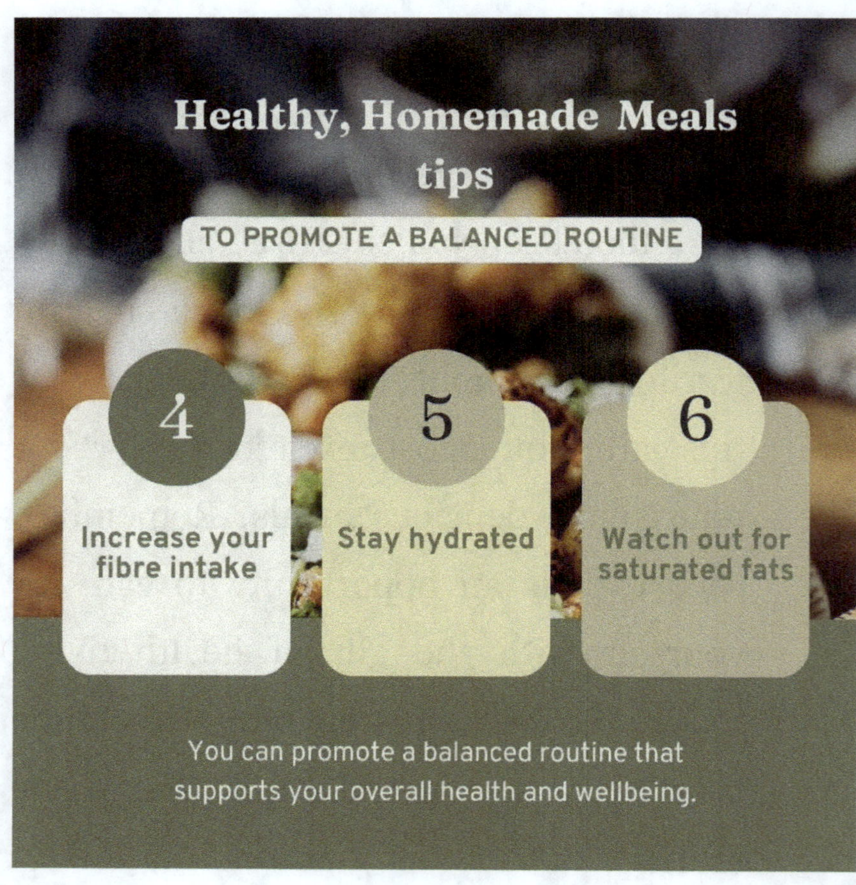

Healthy, Homemade Meals
tips
TO PROMOTE A BALANCED ROUTINE
4
Increase your fibre intake
5
Stay hydrated
6
Watch out for saturated fats
You can promote a balanced routine that supports your overall health and wellbeing.

Chapter 3

DIY Beauty and Grooming

for Self-Care

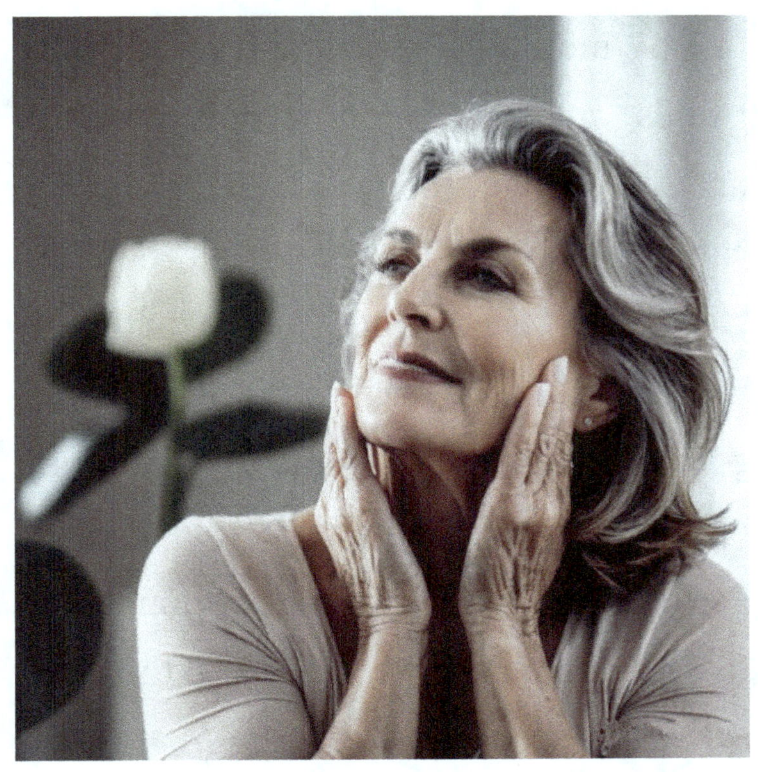

Welcome to Chapter 3, where we'll explore using natural ingredients to nourish ourselves from the outside in through homemade beauty and grooming.

Like many women, I've spent far too much money on the latest skincare trends, makeup palettes, hair products and more over the years. My bathroom cabinets could stock a small Sephora store! But over time, I realized many products contain synthetic fragrances, preservatives and chemicals that don't exactly nurture the body.

Passionate about wellness, I longed to take better care of my body and the earth by using natural, non-toxic beauty products. Commercial products also come with a high price tag! But I struggled to find natural items that performed well at an affordable cost. Then I discovered the joy of creating my own luxurious, effective beauty remedies from simple kitchen ingredients.

DIY beauty is incredibly empowering! With a little kitchen chemistry, you can craft high-quality, customized products that rival department stores find. Using nourishing plant oils, herbs, vitamins and minerals allows you to control exactly what goes on your body. And making your own allows you to adjust recipes perfectly to your skin or hair type.

In this chapter, we'll explore:

- Benefits of natural skincare and ingredients to avoid
- Homemade cleansers, scrubs, masks, creams and serums
- DIY hair masks, shampoos and styling products
- Whipped body butters, sugar scrubs and bath treats
- Natural makeup you can make
- Developing personal style and confidence

Get ready to unleash your inner kitchen cosmetologist! Making your own products is enjoyable, affordable and eco-friendly. These homemade body treats turn self-care into a delightful ritual.

The Benefits of Natural Beauty:

Have you ever actually looked at the tiny list of ingredients on your beauty products? The long, unpronounceable chemical names reveal very little about what's being absorbed into the body. Synthetic fragrances, preservatives, stabilizers, colors and foaming agents have questionable impacts on hormones, neurochemistry and organ function.

For example, the commonly used preservative parabens mimic estrogen in the body, disrupting delicate hormonal balance. Phthalates that enhance texture and flexibility have been tied to reproductive issues and birth defects. Chemical stabilizers penetrate deeply but are difficult for the body to eliminate. The long-term effects of daily exposure are concerning.

Thankfully, we can easily avoid hazardous additives by choosing natural,

non-toxic products – especially by making our own! Common natural ingredients like plant oils, butters and extracts nourish skin gently. Herbs, clays and minerals provide therapeutic benefits without nasty side effects. Homemade products also skip packaging waste and the carbon footprint of shipping.

Seeking out greener beauty swaps protects your body and the planet. You deserve to feel confident that your beauty routine contributes to wellness, not harm. Now let's explore some amazing natural ingredients.

Natural Skincare Ingredients Experimenting with different natural oils, herbs and minerals allows you to create customized products based on your skin type. Here are some of my favorite ingredients for glowing skin:

Base Oils - Sweet almond, coconut, jojoba, avocado, olive and grapeseed oil soften skin and help other ingredients penetrate. Choose according to your preferences and skin type.

Essential Oils - For fragrance, try gentle lavender, uplifting wild orange, refreshing peppermint and tea tree for blemishes. Always dilute oils before applying directly.

Clays - Bentonite and kaolin clays draw out impurities and naturally exfoliate when mixed into masks. French green clay balances oily skin.

Natural Waxes - Beeswax and candelilla wax thicken balms and give lotions a creamy texture without chemicals.

Herbs - Chamomile, calendula and comfrey soothe skin. Turmeric, neem and gout kola ease inflammation. Thyme and rosemary cleanse.

Vitamin E - Found in oils like wheat germ and sunflower seed, vitamin E is anti-aging, hydrating and healing for skin.

Minerals - Bentonite clay, magnesium flakes and colloidal oatmeal strengthen and nourish skin.

With endless combinations, you can create personalized cleansers, scrubs, masks, moisturizers and more! Now let's get to recipes...

Homemade Facial Cleanser

Gentle oil cleansing melts away makeup, sunscreen and impurities without stripping skin. The nourishing oils won't disrupt your natural moisture barrier like harsh foaming cleansers.

Combine the following in a glass bottle and shake before each use:

- 1/2 cup carrier oil like jojoba, grapeseed or sunflower
- 1/4 cup castor oil, which helps remove stubborn makeup
- 10 drops tea tree, lavender or geranium essential oil

To use: Massage 1-2 tsp all over dry face and neck in circular motions. Rinse with a warm, wet washcloth then splash face with cool water to tighten pores. Store cleanser in the fridge if your skin tends to be oily.

Exfoliating Face Scrub

Slough away dull cells for fresh, glowy skin using this invigorating homemade scrub a few times per week. The gentle exfoliants won't tear skin like harsh micro-beads.

Mix the following in a small bowl:

- 2 tablespoons coarse sugar or fine oats
- 1 tablespoon raw honey to help bind ingredients
- 1 tablespoon olive, almond or jojoba oil
- 5 drops lavender, lemon or grapefruit essential oil

Gently massage over damp skin, rinse and finish with a splash of cool water to tighten pores. Limit use to 2-3 times a week to avoid over-exfoliating.

Hydrating Sheet Mask

This nourishing soak infuses moisture into dry or dull skin for an instant pick-me-up. The gelatin powder firms as it dries to keep potent ingredients pressed against skin.

In a bowl, mix:

- 1 tablespoon unflavored gelatin powder
- 1 cup boiling water
- 1 teaspoon honey
- 1 tablespoon apple cider vinegar
- Optional: mashed avocado, aloe vera gel or finely ground oats Allow

to cool slightly then soak cotton rounds or a cloth face mask in the mixture. Apply to clean your face and relax 10-15 minutes before rinsing. Keep unused portions refrigerated for another use.

Clarifying Clay Mask

Clays absorb excess oil, draw out impurities and reduce inflammation or acne. This medicinal mask leaves skin clear, smooth and balanced.

Stir together:

- 2 tablespoons bentonite, French green or kaolin clay
- 1 tablespoon raw honey

- 1 teaspoon apple cider vinegar or lemon juice
- Enough water to form spreadable paste

Apply to damp skin, avoiding eye area. Allow to dry 15 minutes before rinsing clean. Use 1-2 times per week for clear, vibrant skin.

Anti-Aging Serum

Plump skin and minimize fine lines with this silky, nutrient-dense serum. The antioxidants and essential fatty acids promote collagen production and hydration.

In a small bottle or jar, combine:

- ¼ cup pomegranate seed oil or sea buckthorn oil, which are high in wrinkle-fighting antioxidants

- 1 tablespoon rosehip oil to boost collagen

- ½ teaspoon vitamin E oil to strengthen skin

- 5 drops frankincense essential oil, which has anti-aging properties

Use morning and night after cleansing. Warm a few drops in palms and gently pat into skin. Store unused serum in the fridge.

Soothing Eye Cream

Thin skin around the eyes needs special

care. Chamomile, vitamin E and plant oils in this blend reduce puffiness, hydrates and protects against environmental damage.

Whisk together:

- 1 tablespoon of jojoba or coconut, olive oil

- ½ teaspoon beeswaxpellets to thicken

- ½ teaspoon almond, sunflower or vitamin E oil

- ½ teaspoon chamomile hydrosol or strong chilled tea

- 5 drops chamomile essential oil

Warm in fingers before gently dabbing around the eye area morning and night. Store in the fridge between uses.

Natural Haircare DIY

Just like skin, our hair deserves nourishing ingredients free of sulfates, silicone and synthetic fragrances. Treat your lovely locks to these natural spa-inspired formulas.

Soothing Aloe & Honey Hair Mask This hydrating treatment smooth and softens for shiny, manageable locks.

Combine in a bowl:

- ¼ cup fresh aloe Vera gel, which contains enzymes that repair damage
- ¼ cup coconut oil to strengthen and protect
- 1 tablespoon raw honey to seal in moisture

- 10 drops lavender or rosemary essential oil for a pleasant scent

Shampoo hair then work the mask thoroughly. Pile hair into a shower cap and let sit for 30 minutes. Rinse out in the shower. Use 1-2 times per week.

Clarifying Apple Cider Vinegar Rinse

This gentle rinse removes buildup, balances pH and adds shine for healthy hair and scalp.

After shampooing, slowly pour the following through clean, wet hair:

- 1 cup warm water

- 2 tablespoons apple cider vinegar

- 5 drops tea tree or rosemary essential oil (optional) Massage into the scalp and comb through the hair. Let sit 1-2 minutes before rinsing out. Use 1-2 times per week.

Valorizing Dry Shampoo

Refresh limp hair by absorbing oil with this simple dry shampoo you can make for pennies.

Mix the following in a salt or pepper shaker:

- 3 tablespoons cornstarch or arrowroot powder

- 1 tablespoon cocoa powder for darker hair, or leave out for light hair
- 10 drops essential oil like grapefruit or lemon (optional)

Shake powder through roots and work in with fingers to absorb oil. Style as desired. Shake off excess.

Defrizzing Hair Serum

Tame unruly frizz and flyaway while adding shine and silkiness with regular use of this serum.

Combine in a spray bottle or glass dropper bottle:

- 1/4 cup coconut, argon or jojoba oil
- 2 tablespoons aloe Vera gel

- 1 tablespoon vitamin E oil

- 10 drops lavender essential oil

Apply a few drops while hair is still damp before blow-drying or air drying. Focus on ends and flyways.

With these natural formulations, you can recreate the salon experience at home! Now let's shift focus to body care products.

DIY Body Care Recipes

Your body's largest organ deserves the very best care for optimal health. When you make your own body lotions, scrubs and bath products, you know exactly what's being absorbed. These recipes are

simple to whip up in your kitchen.
Natural Body Butter Bar

This solid moisturizer glides over skin, leaving it supple and nourished. Bars are perfect for dry hands and feet but can be used all over.

Melt together in a double boiler:

- 1⁄4 cup mango, cocoa or shea butter
  - 1⁄4 cup coconut or sweet almond oil
- 1 tablespoon beeswax Once melted and combined, pour into silicone molds or a loaf pan lined with parchment paper. Allow to cool completely before using. Apply as needed to soften and hydrate skin.

Fizzy Bath Bombs

Pamper yourself with these effervescent bath bombs that moisturize while releasing essential oils.
Mix the following in a large bowl:

- 2 cups baking soda

- 1 cup cornstarch

- 1/4 cup citric acid

- 2 tablespoons Epsom salts

- 1 teaspoon olive, coconut or almond oil

- 10-15 drops essential oils like eucalyptus or lavender

Slowly spritz the surface with witch hazel or aloe vera gel until clumps form. Pack tightly into molds and allow to dry overnight before using.

Citrus Sugar Body Scrub

Invigorate dull skin with this naturally exfoliating scrub sweetened with orange essential oil.

Stir together:

- ½ cup fine granulated sugar

- ¼ cup coconut or olive oil

- Zest of 1 orange or grapefruit

- 10 drops sweet orange essential oil Gently massage over damp skin while showering. Rinse clean. Store leftover scrub in the fridge between uses.

Whipped Body Butter

This velvety cream melts into skin, sealing in softness and moisture all day long.

Using a stand mixer, whip together:

- ½ cup coconut oil

- ¼ cup shea or cocoa butter

- 1 tablespoon honey

- 1 teaspoon vitamin E oil

- 10 drops essential oil like lavender Once light and fluffy, store the body butter in the fridge or freezer.

Apply after bathing or showering to lock in hydration.

Take time to care for your whole body with these soothing homemade treats.

Next let's explore makeup!

Natural Makeup You Can Make

Commercial makeup often contains talc, synthetic dyes and other questionable fillers. But the good news is many cosmetics can be made at home using healthy ingredients. Get creative with these ideas!

Tinted Lip Balm – Blend 1 tablespoon beeswax, 2 tablespoons coconut or almond oil and a dash of natural color from berries, beet powder or cocoa powder. Pour into chopstick tubes or a small tin.

Mineral Blush — Finely grind red or pink clay in a mortar and pestle or blender. Mix with a few teaspoons of arrowroot powder or cornstarch. Apply with a makeup brush.

Mascara — Activate 1 tablespoon activated charcoal powder with 1 teaspoon aloe Vera gel. Use a clean mascara wand to brush through lashes.

Eyeshadow — Make loose powder eyeshadow by micronizing cosmetic clay or cocoa powder in a blender. Press into the pan of an old eyeshadow compact. **Concealer** – Mix 1/2 teaspoon bentonite clay with 1 tablespoon coconut oil. Add zinc oxidepowder to lighten or yellow oxide for golden tones. Use on spotsor under eyes. With simple ingredients from nature, you can make quality cosmetics customized to your coloring and preferences. Now let's explore elevating your personal style.

Developing Your Signature Style

Outer beauty radiates from self-confidence and loving yourself as you are. But expressing your personal style can definitely help you feel more comfortable in your skin. When you dress in clothes that align with your values and sensibilities, inner beauty shines through. Here are tips for cultivating a wardrobe and beauty routine that feels authentic:

- Collect inspiration images of styles and looks you admire to find trends that appeal to you.
- Determine your color season to select hues that complement your complexion, hair and eyes.
- Identify your body type and learn which silhouettes and lines are most flattering.
- Take inventory of your current closet and makeup. Look for gaps and redundancies.

- Invest in quality over quantity, focusing on versatile basics in fabrics that feel nice.

- Include comfortable yet polished lounge- and workout-wear.

- Incorporate pops of color and accessorize to reflect your personality.

- Play with new makeup techniques when you're in the mood for fun.

- Wear what makes YOU smile when you look in the mirror.

When you identify a style that aligns with your essence, getting dressed and ready each day becomes an enjoyable creative ritual of self-expression. You'll glow with confidence in clothes that fit your body and personality.

In closing, I hope this chapter inspired you to see beauty and grooming as opportunities for self-care and creative expression. With nourishing natural ingredients and a signature look aligned with your spirit, outer radiance will mirror your inner light. Here's to embracing your unique beauty, perfectly imperfections and all!

I make my health and self-care a priority each day.

I flourish when I nurture my mind, body and spirit.

My journey of self-care awakens joy and vitality.

I lovingly care for my whole self – I am worth it!

I embrace each moment and stage of life with grace.

DIY BEAUTY AND GROOMING

for Self-Care

Shave regularly. You don't want to look like a grungy mess all day long. Also wash your hair twice a week Make sure your hair is properly styled and trimmed

Clean your face and neck daily.

Use a moisturiser every day. Moisturisers help keep your skin supple and hydrated, which helps reduce the appearance of wrinkles and lines.

Look for products that are made with natural ingredients. Natural ingredients are better for your skin and they won't cause any irritation or allergies.

Lilly Green

Lilly Green

Chapter 4

Lifelong Wellness for Women

Before we dive into tips to support women's health and wellbeing, allow me to share a funny story that taught me an important self-care lesson.

In my late 20s, I worked long hours climbing the corporate ladder as a marketing manager. I barely made time to eat, let alone schedule a check-up. I figured at my age, I was invincible anyway. So I skipped my annual women's health exam for nearly 3 years straight.

Not smart, I know!

Finally, one October I decided I was overdue for a pap smear and breast exam. I booked an appointment and went in, embarrassed to admit how long it had been. The compassionate nurse practitioner said not to worry, they were just glad to see me taking charge of my health.

As I got settled on the exam table in that paper gown, she made small talk asking if I had big Halloween plans. I mentioned my waitress costume, feeling a bit silly at my age. She assured me it's healthy to get in touch with your inner child sometimes!

Right on cue, I cracked up laughing at that phrase just as she inserted the speculum for my pap smear. My sudden burst of laughter at that inopportune moment startled the poor NP, who also started giggling. There we both sat chuckling away hysterically in the exam room.

Though uncomfortable, we managed to finish the exam while giggling. She reminded me to schedule annual women's visits going forward. I left feeling grateful not just for compassionate care, but the reminder not to take myself too seriously.

While maintaining health is serious business, joy and laughter are equally vital. In this chapter, we'll cover all aspects of lifelong wellness for women while making room for humor too. Let's get started!

The Importance of Self-Care

A famous saying goes "You can't pour from an empty cup." Yet as women, we often deplete our own wellbeing striving to care for others - as partners, mothers, daughters, employees and more. When we run on empty, everything suffers including our ability to show up.

Self-care allows your cup to remain full. Taking time to nurture body and soul proactively prevents depletion and burnout. You gain energy to care for loved ones whilemodeling healthy habits. Self-care benefits everyone!

But what does self-care actually entail? It's more than weekly bubble baths and massages (although those are wonderful too!). Ongoing self-care practices help you thrive in all aspects of health:

- Physical - nourishing diet, exercise, medical care, rest
- Mental - managing stress, boundaries, social connections
- Emotional - processing feelings, self-compassion, counseling
- Spiritual - practices like meditation, journaling, nature time
- Financial - wise budgeting, debt management, retirement savings

When all aspects of your wellbeing are nourished, you create a solid foundation for weathering life's joys and challenges from a place of strength. Let's explore specific ways to care for health at every age.

Wellness in Your 20s

Our 20s are filled with exploration and change as we build careers, relationships and independence. It's an ideal time to establish self-care habits that serve you for life. Here are wellness tips for thriving in your 20s:

- Stay active with sports or classes for strong bones, muscles and heart health

- Fuel your body with nutrient-dense foods to maintain energy and
mental clarity Visit a gynecologist each year for reproductive health exams and STI testing

- Create time for hobbies, interests and friendship amidst your busy schedule

- Get 7-9 hours of quality sleep nightly to manage stress and

Consolidate learning

- Talk to a therapist or counselor if you struggle with anxiety,

Depression or stress

• Take time for self-reflection through journaling, meditation or contemplative walking

Save consistently each month, even if just a little, to start financial plannin boundaries around work, technology and perfectionism to avoid burnout

Your 20s are meant for exploration, learning and growth. Make self-care a priority now to set positive patterns that sustain you for decades to come.

Wellness in Your 30s

Your 30s see many women settling into careers, long-term relationships and new family roles. It's a prime time to develop self-care practices that help you balance thriving in all areas.

Get proper sleep to keep up with likely busier schedule and responsibilities

- Hydrate with water and nutrient-rich foods to maintain preconception health
- Take time to move your body with walks, prenatal yoga if pregnant, and pelvic floor exercises
- Make your annual well-woman exam for reproductive health screenings
- Surround yourself with supportive friends and family you can rely on

- Set boundaries around work and obligations to prevent burnout
  Reflect through journaling on identity, purpose and what brings joy
- Budget wisely as expenses grow, saving what you can for the future
- Make space for your relationship amidst parenting, caring for your partnership
- Find humor and laughter in the chaos of juggling family and career

Balancing expanded responsibilities in your 30s isn't easy, but self-care ensures you continue prioritizing YOU while giving to others.

Wellness in Your 40s

Your 40s open a time of reflection on how to live your best life. It's normal for Priorities and health needs to shift as we age. Adjust your self-care practices accordingly with these tips:

• Schedule mammograms and bone density tests as recommended

• Incorporate strength training and impact exercise for metabolism and bone health

- Sustain energy and brain health with a Mediterranean style diet high in omega-3s

- Make time for pelvic floor physical therapy if needed for bladder leaks or prolapse
  - Talk with your doctor about perimenopause symptoms if your periods change
  - Connect with friends who inspire and uplift you through shared interests

- Find work that aligns with your values if you desire career changes

- Make plans for retirement and evaluate current financial standing

- Practice self-compassion and set boundaries around self-criticism

- Explore complementary therapies like acupuncture if you experience joint pain or sleep issues Your 40s highlight the importance of nurturing mental and spiritual well being alongside physical health. Self-care now sets you up for your most vibrant chapter yet!

Wellness in Your 50s and Beyond

There is so much beauty to be embraced in midlife and beyond! Stay empowered navigating changes like menopause and aging with proper self-care:

- Maintain health screenings like mammograms and colonoscopies
- Incorporate cardio and strength training into your exercise routine -Fuel your body with extra calcium, vitamin D and antioxidants
- Make vaginal health a priority if you experience dryness or discomfort
- Treat hot flashes, sleep disruption and low moods related to

menopause

Volunteer or take a class to meet
new people and engage your mind

- Retire debt, downsize if desired and
refine your estate planning

- Explore your spiritual side through
practices like meditation or
journaling

- Have compassion for yourself and
release the pressure of
perfectionism

- Express your vibrant, wise and
passionate inner spirit! Caring for
your wellbeing helps you embrace
midlife and beyond with grace.
Remember, self-care is a lifelong

process, not a singular destination. Adjust practices as life evolves while honoring your basic needs.

Now let's talk about balance!

Achieving Wellness Balance

Here's the thing about self-care - it's all about balance! Too little, and we deplete our reserves. Too much, and we become self-absorbed. True wellbeing arises when we nurture ourselves while also giving to others and the world around us. I like to visualize my responsibilities and self-care practices as colorful mosaic tiles. Each one has its own shape and hue. Some days, certain tiles may dominate as I spend more time on work, family or rest. But over the long-term, I aim to create an even mosaic with self-care routines woven throughout each day. Proper balance looks different for everyone since we all have unique priorities and needs. Reflect on how you can best integrate the following elements:

- Nourishing basics like healthy food, hydration and sleep
- Household and family care like chores, child-rearing and pet time
- Professional passion through purposeful work or education
- Physical activity for strength, cardio and enjoyment
- Creative outlets that spark joy and relaxation
- Down time where you simply rest and recharge
- Social connections that energize and inspire you

Mindfully craft each day to incorporate care for yourself and others. Savor moments of connection and joy amidst obligations. Establish routines while allowing flexibility when needed. Seek progress, not perfection each day.

When you feel like the balance shifts too far to one extreme, make adjustments. Cut back if self-care veers toward indulgence. Speak up if you take on too much. Balance takes practice, but the payoff is serenity and lasting contentment. In closing, I hope this chapter provided motivation to keep self-care and joyful wellbeing at the heart of your days, decades and life path ahead. Remember to show up fully for others only once your own cup is full. Make your health a priority - body, mind and spirit. Stay open and optimistic as each chapter unfolds. Most importantly, greet yourself and each new day with patience, understanding and compassion. Here's to wellness from the inside out!

Bonus Chapter

Everyday Wellness for Women

As we conclude our wellness journey together, I wanted to share a bonus tips focused on practical self-care tools you can start implementing today. While long bubble baths and beach vacations sound nice, real life demands simple practices that fit into regular routines.

The good news is that small, consistent self-care actions often have the greatest impact. Like compound interest, the benefits accumulate over time to create deep positive change. Let's explore tangible ways to support thriving in five key areas: sleep, exercise, women's health, social connections and self-compassion.

Optimizing Sleep for Better Days Ahead The saying "make time to sleep, or you'll have to make time for illness" rings so true. When we short-change our body's need for restoration, everything suffers. Yet busy schedules and anxiety often rob us of quality sleep. How can we make the most of our time in bed?

My friend Alicia is a sleep expert who transformed my own sleeping habits. She explains that preparing your mindset, environment and routine for optimal rest makes all the difference. Here are some of her top tips that helped me go from tossing and turning to sound slumber each night:

- Keep a consistent bedtime and wake time, even on weekends
- Avoid screens, big meals and stimulating tasks before bedtime
- Create an ideal cool, dark, quiet sleep sanctuary
- Spend the hour before bed reading, stretching or meditating
- Let worries go by jotting concerns in a journal before lights out
- Use a white noise machine or app if ambient noise disrupts you

- Consider blackout curtains if early morning light awakens you

- Talk to your doctor if insomnia, hot flashes or apnea persist Now I follow a soothing pre-bed routine that cues my body that it's time for rest. Aim for 7-9 hours of quality sleep regularly to energize each day. Your mind and body will thank you.

IntegratingMovementforEnergyand Strength

Like many women, my exercise habits have ebbed and flowed over the years with busy seasons of life. But my friend Julia taught me that consistent movement, even just a little, changes everything.

As a mom and small business owner, Julia struggled to find the time and motivation for structured workouts. She'd do well for a month or two, then fall off the exercise wagon as her hectic schedule took over. It became an all-or-nothing cycle of starting and stopping that often left her discouraged. What finally worked was integrating motion into her daily routines. Now Julia simply looks for opportunities to move a few minutes here and there. She shared some examples that have made a huge difference:

- Doing squats or lunges during kitchen clean-up or brushing her teeth
- Using a standing desk or taking hourly movement breaks when working
- Walking her son to and from the bus stop each morning and afternoon
- Doing five minutes of stretches while watching TV after dinner
- Parking farther away at stores to get extra walking time
- Taking the stairs whenever possible for a quick burst activity Julia's whole mindset shifted from finding big chunks of workout time to

simply moving more all day long. Even 10-15 minutes sprinkled throughout your routine keeps your energy and metabolism humming. Look for moments to include activities you enjoy! Proactively Caring for Women's Health Earlier in the book, I shared my funny story about delaying my annual well-woman exam for several years when I was in my late twenties. Sound familiar to anyone?

While there's nothing fun about pap smears or mammograms, I learned the importance of taking charge of my reproductive and overall health through regular preventative care. My friend

Tracey, a OB-GYN nurse practitioner, offers this helpful perspective:

"I know exams, tests and shots sound less than appealing. But just remember screening and vaccines allow us to detect issues early or even prevent them altogether. Living life to the fullest means being proactive so you CAN keep living your best life! Stay on top of:

- Annual well-woman visit including Pap, breast exam, STI testing

- Regular mammograms once you hit 40, or earlier if high risk

- HPV vaccine if under 45 to prevent cervical cancer

- Colonoscopies every 5-10 years beginning at 45, and earlier if risk factors
- Bone density testing at 65 plus getting enough calcium and vitamin D
- Pelvic health: Kegels, physical therapy, hormone therapy if needed Pair clinical care with lifestyle pillars like nutrition, exercise, stress relief and community for whole woman support." Thanks to Tracey, I now keep up with important health visits that used to make me cringe. Protecting wellbeing begins with self-care like exams. You've got this, ladies!

The Healing Power of Community

Remember that saying "Joy shared is joy multiplied?" I've found that to be so true when making meaningful connections. But amidst busy seasons, it's easy to unintentionally isolate just when you need uplifting community most.

My friend Renee moved to a new city right before the pandemic hit. While working remotely, she struggled to establish her "people" locally outside of her partner. When everything reopened, she committed to putting herself out there.

Here are some of the strategies that worked for Renee:

- She joined a recreational soccer team to meet friends with a shared interest.

- She hosted a potluck dinner and invited co-workers she wanted to get to know better.

- She volunteered once a week at a women's shelter, sensing it would fill her cup too.

- She signed up for a watercolor painting class that piqued her creativity.

- She adopted a dog knowing it would get her walking and conversing around the neighborhood.

As Renee watered the seeds of connection, she created a blossoming sense of belonging. She realized wellness comes not just from eating right and exercise, but laughing with others who light up your soul.

Nurture your social wellness by reaching out to kindred spirits and contributing your gifts. Don't underestimate the heart-healing power of a community.

Self-Compassion for Stressful Times

When this book was originally conceived pre-pandemic, I never could have imagined the intense stress and chaos that would unfold. It's been a deeply unsettling time full of difficult emotions like grief, fear and uncertainty. What has helped me remain grounded through it all is self-compassion.

My therapist often reminds me to talk to myself as I would a dear friend in need of support. We would never shame a friend for feeling vulnerable during hard times. So why judge yourself?

Here are little ways I show myself extra gentleness and care:

- Saying "this is really tough right now, let me comfort and nourish myself."
- Taking a pause to breathe deeply when I feel anxious or overwhelmed.
- Getting outside in nature daily for a fresh perspective.

- Letting go of perfectionism around work and parenting. We're all doing our best.

- Following my body's need for rest when I feel depleted. Things can wait.

- Surrounding myself with hopeful, positive people. Limit time with those who drain you.

- Remembering "this too shall pass" and looking for positive signs of progress.

While self-care keeps your tank full, self-compassion reminds you to be gentle when you inevitably feel drained or stuck. Speak to yourself as a caring friend. Together we'll get through this. In closing, I hope this bonus tips provided helpful, bite-sized wellness inspiration you can apply immediately.

Small consistent actions tailored to your needs make all the difference. Prioritize sleep, hydration, nutrition and movement.

Seek support when needed. Most importantly, care for your whole being with compassion you deserve   it!

Wishing you continued health, wisdom and joy ahead

Conclusion

As we conclude our wellness journey together, remember that self-care is a lifelong practice with immense rewards when maintained over time. Start where you are, honor your needs, release judgment and be consistent. Small actions accumulate to create deep nourishment and balance of body and spirit. Trust your inner wisdom to craft a self-care routine that fits your life. You deserve to feel empowered in your health, relationships, work and beyond. May you continue to care for your beautiful self with compassion. Wishing you continued growth, wisdom and wellbeing in the days ahead!

Index

Introduction

The Author

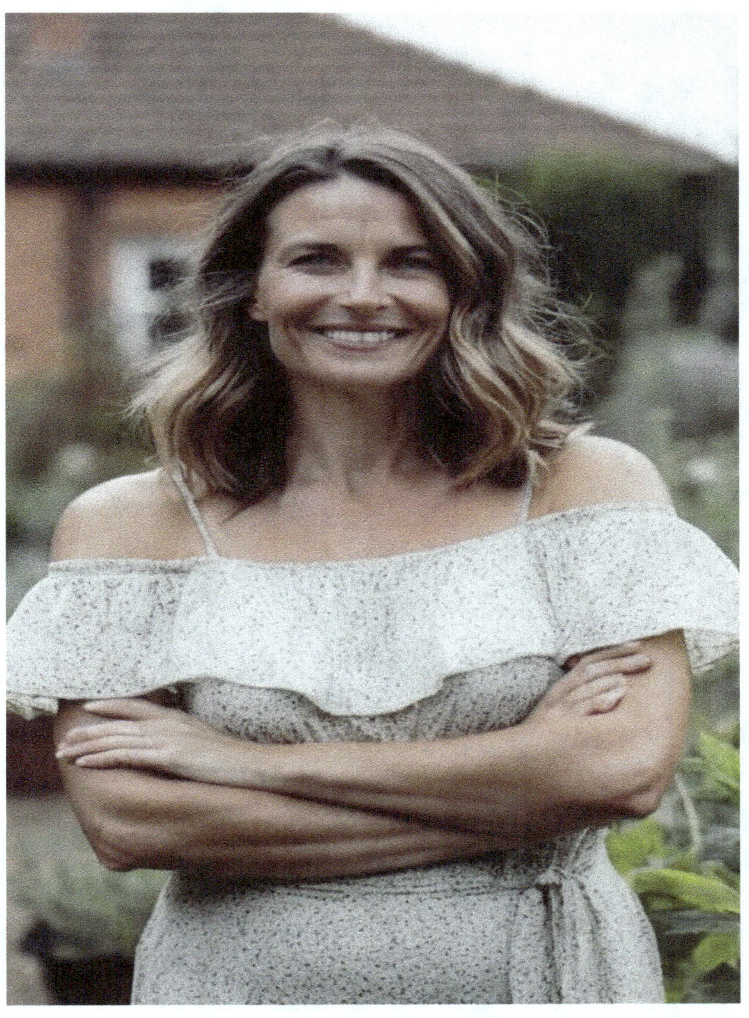